@RosenTeenTalk

AUTISM

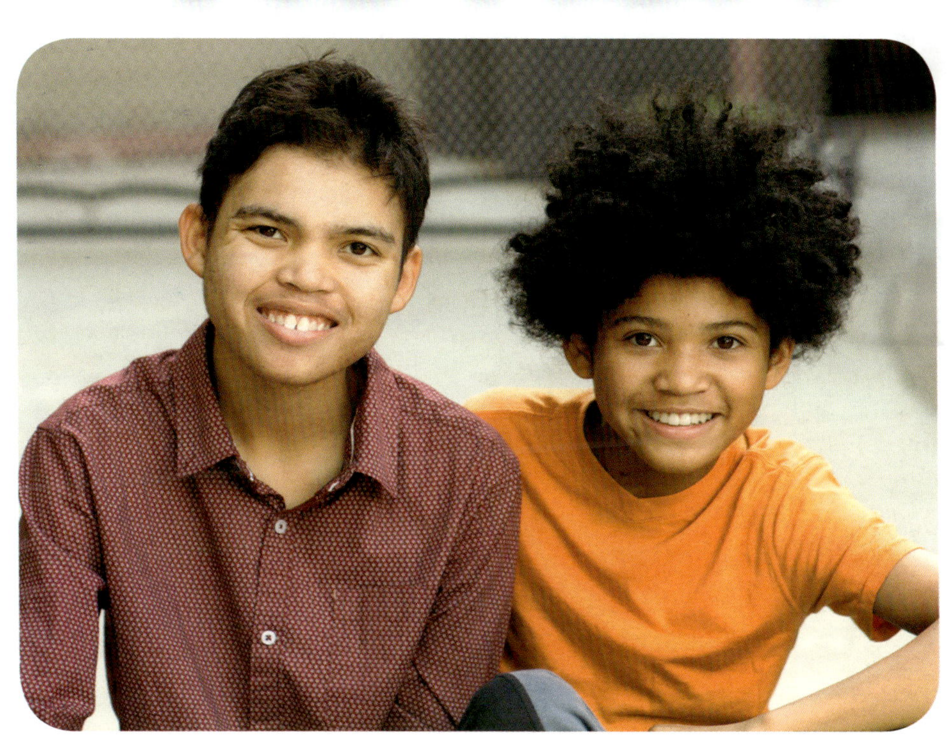

Stephane Hillard

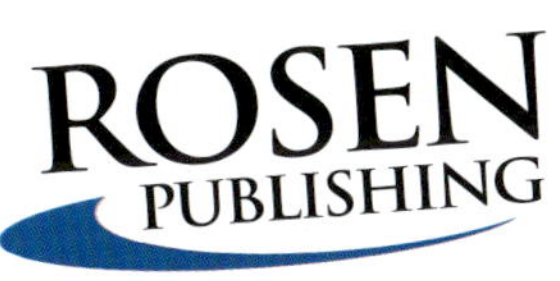

ROSEN PUBLISHING
NEW YORK

Published in 2021 by The Rosen Publishing Group, Inc.
29 East 21st Street, New York, NY 10010

First Edition

Editor: Theresa Emminizer
Designer: Michael Flynn
Interior Layout: Rachel Rising

Photo Credits: Cover, pp. 3, 4, 45 pixelheadphoto digitalskillet/Shutterstock.com; Cover Denis Gorelkin/Shutterstock.com; Cover, pp. 1, 6, 8, 10, 12, 16, 18, 20, 24, 26, 28, 30, 32, 36, 38, 40, 42 Vitya_M/Shutterstock.com; pp. 3, 15 martinedoucet/ E+/Getty Images; pp. 3, 23 BSIP / Contributor/ Universal Images Group/Getty Images; pp. 3, 35 Jerod Harris / Stringer/ Getty Images North America/Getty Images; pp. 6, 30 wallybird/Shutterstock.com; p. 7 vetre/ Shutterstock.com; p. 8 Mark J Hunt/Getty Images; p. 9 Image taken by Mayte Torres/ Moment/Getty Images; p. 11 SolStock/E+/Getty Images; p. 12 Daniel Boczarski / Stringer/ Getty Images North America/Getty Images; p. 13 Yeexin Richelle/Shutterstock.com; p. 16 FatCamera/E+/Getty Images; p, 17 Dmytro Zinkevych/ Shutterstock.com; p. 19 Marol/Shutterstock.com; p. 20 pagadesign/E+/Getty Images; p. 21 Frank Calleja / Contributor/ Toronto Star/Getty Images; p. 24 Jonathan Leibson / Stringer/ Getty Images Entertainment/Getty Images; p. 25 nakaridore/Shutterstock.com; p. 26 H.S. Photos / Alamy Stock Photo; p. 27 Pixel-Shot/Shutterstock.com; p. 28 SDI Productions/E+/Getty Images; p. 29 Andy Sacks/ The Image Bank/Getty Images; p. 31 Daisy Daisy/Shutterstock.com; p. 32 Thomas Andre Fure/Shutterstock.com; p. 33 Photographee.eu/Shutterstock.com; p. 36 hidesy/Shutterstock.com; p.37 Araya Diaz / Contributor/ Getty Images Entertainment/Getty Images; p. 38 Rommel Canlas/Shutterstock.com; p. 39 Matej Kastelic/ Shutterstock.com; p.40 artskvortsova/Shutterstock.com; p. 41 Kathy Hutchins/Shutterstock.com; p. 43 Chicago Tribune /Contributor/ Tribune News Service/Getty Images.

Library of Congress Cataloging-in-Publication Data

Names: Hillard, Stephane, author.
Title: Autism / Stephane Hillard.
Description: New York : Rosen Publishing, [2021] | Series: @Rosenteentalk | Includes index.
Identifiers: LCCN 2020012482 | ISBN 9781499467970 (paperback) | ISBN 9781499467987 (library binding)
Subjects: LCSH: Autism spectrum disorders. | Autism in adolescence.
Classification: LCC RC553.A88 H555 2021 | DDC 616.85/882--dc23
LC record available at https://lccn.loc.gov/2020012482

Manufactured in the United States of America

CPSIA Compliance Information: Batch #BSR20. For further information contact Rosen Publishing, New York, New York at 1-800-237-9932.

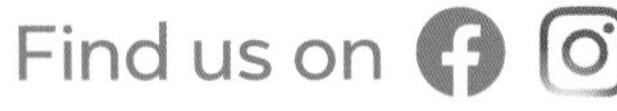

CONTENTS

Chapter 1

Adam's Last First Day

Today was my first day of high school. But, instead of making new friends, I spent my first day worrying about my older brother Adam. Today was Adam's last first day of high school. He's in 12th grade.

Adam has autism spectrum **disorder**, or ASD. He learns differently from most students. He also acts differently from most kids. In school, Adam has a teacher's aide. She helps him stay focused and works with him on **communication** skills. When I was younger, I didn't know why Adam acted differently. My parents explained that even though Adam has ASD, he still has likes and dislikes just like everyone else. I'm worried about what Adam will do after he graduates. Will he get into college or get a job?

Adam has a hard time communicating with others. He also has a hard time understanding why people do the things they do.

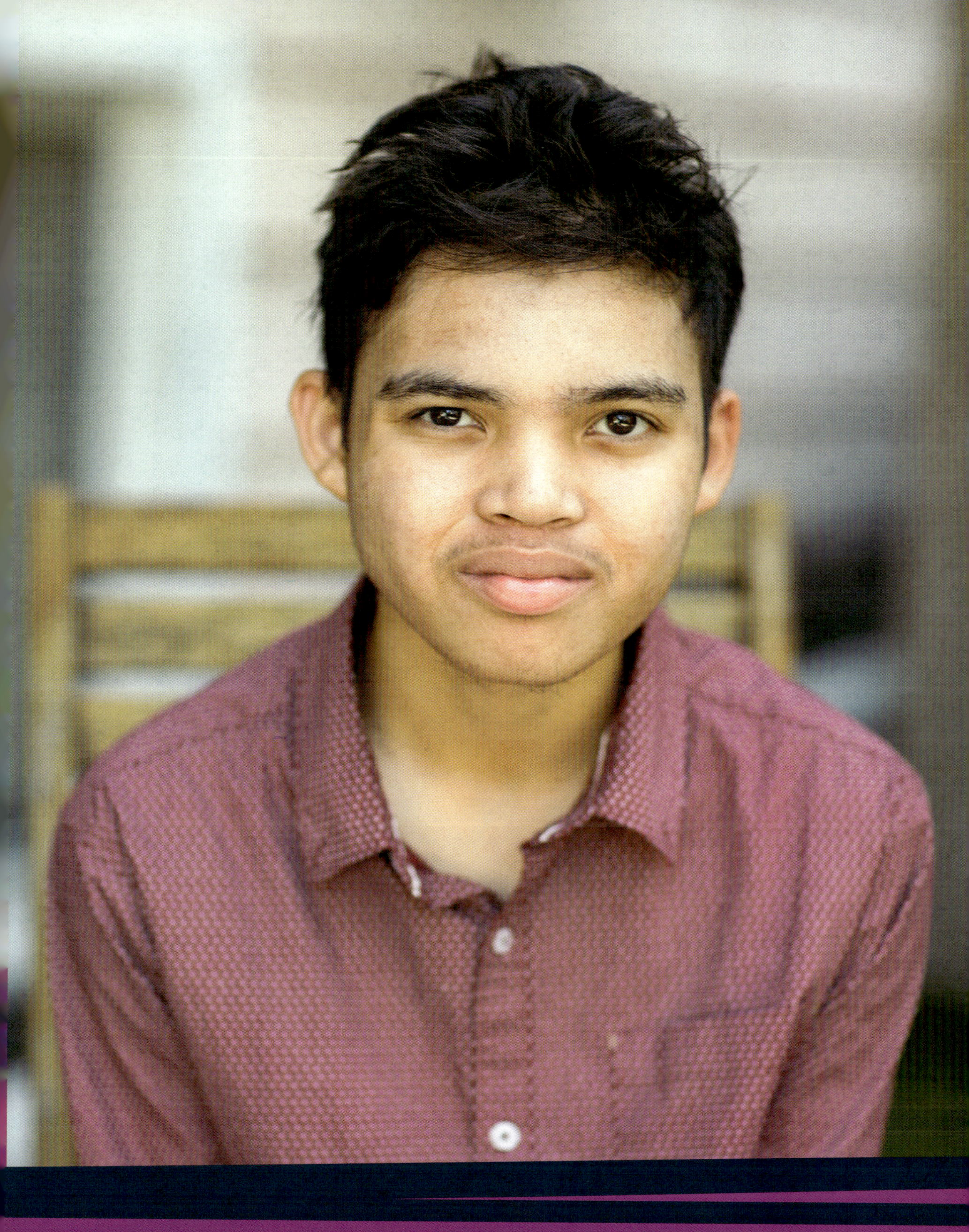

WHAT IS ASD?

ASD is a **developmental** disorder. That means that people who have ASD have **delayed** development. They may be slower to learn, talk, or walk. However, it's a spectrum disorder. That means everyone with ASD is different.

People with ASD don't look any different from other people. ASD can affect all sorts of people. There isn't a cure for ASD. But treatments can make people with ASD feel better. Treatments make it easier for them to do things.

About 44 percent of children with ASD are just as smart or smarter than their peers.

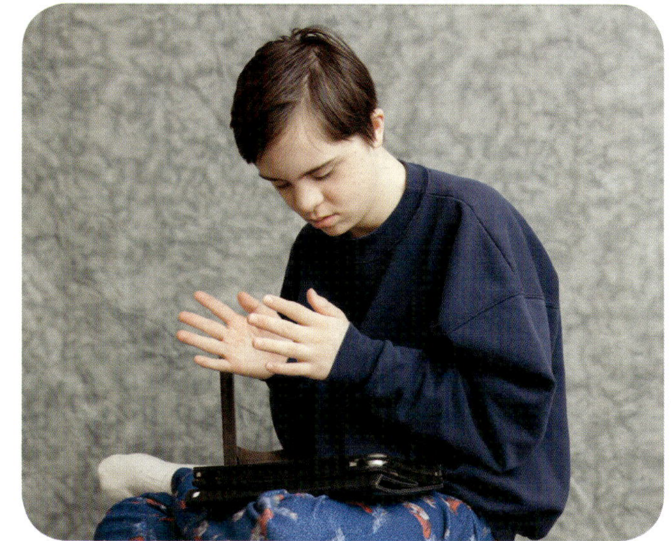

Fast Facts

- **About 1 in 59 children have ASD.**
- **Boys are four times more likely to have ASD than girls.**
- **In about 36 to 95 percent of cases, both identical twins have ASD.**
- **In about 0 to 31 percent of cases, both fraternal twins have ASD.**

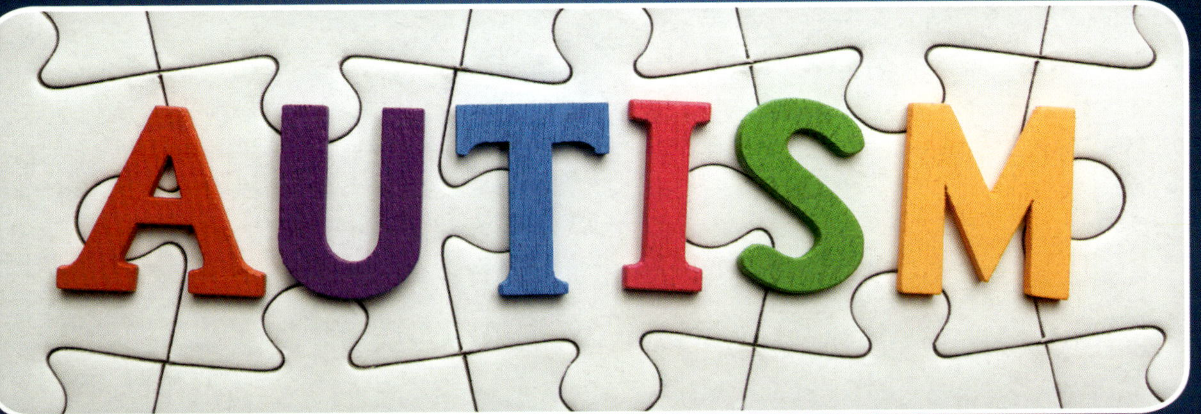

SIGNS OF ASD

Someone with ASD may show one or more of the following signs:

- Trouble talking and communicating
- Repeating words or movements over and over again
- Trouble **adapting** to changes in **routine**
- Doesn't look people in the eye
- Doesn't play "pretend" games

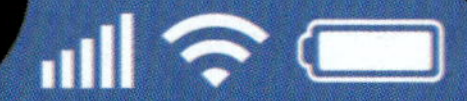

HOW IS ASD DIAGNOSED?

When you go to the doctor, they might test your blood or do an X-ray to **diagnose** you. But that's not how doctors diagnose someone with ASD. To diagnose someone with ASD, doctors have to watch how the person acts and check their development.

It's hard to diagnose adults with ASD. That's because many of ASD's symptoms, or signs, are similar to symptoms of other mental health disorders.

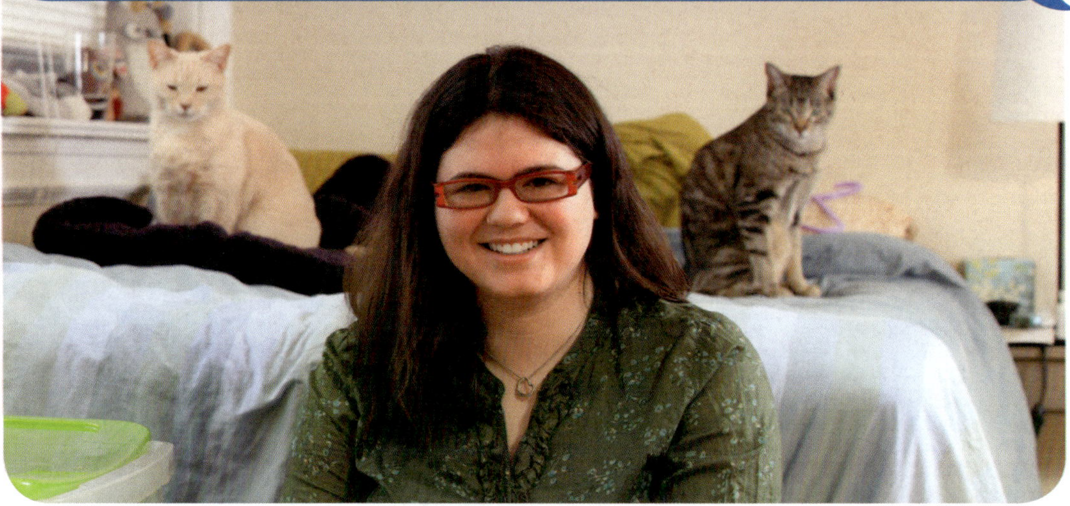

Some people are diagnosed with ASD as young as two years old. Others might not be diagnosed until they're older. The earlier a child is diagnosed with ASD, the more help they can receive.

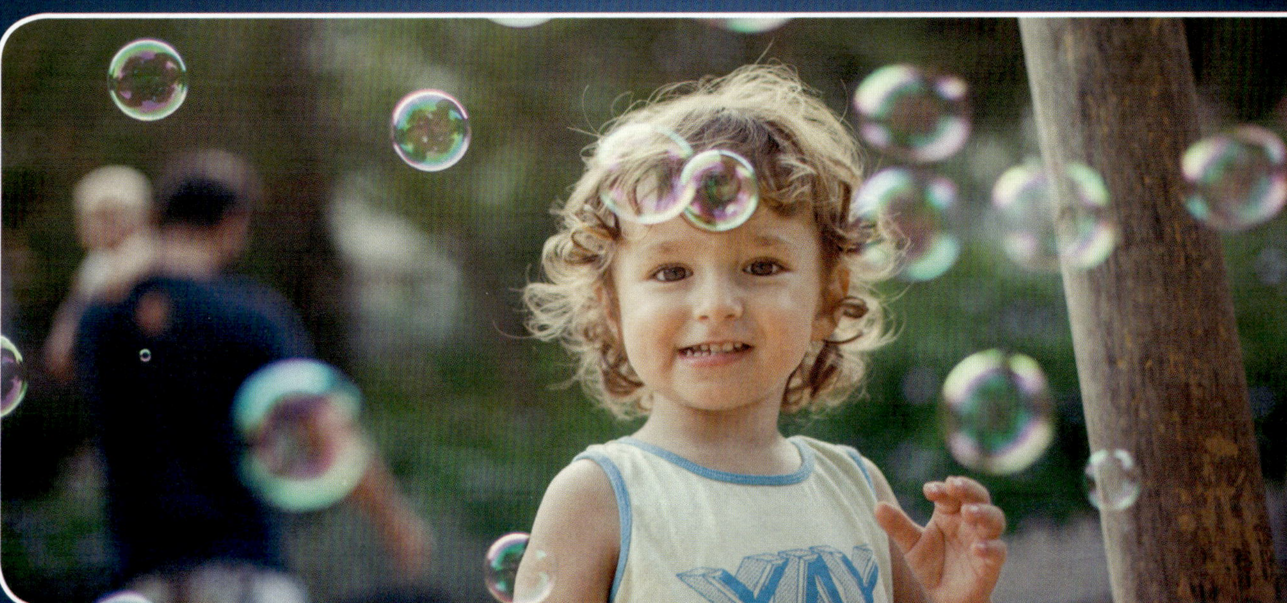

DIFFERENT DIAGNOSES

People with ASD are diagnosed in different ways depending on their age. Young children are diagnosed in two steps. The first happens when they go to the doctor for check-ups. The doctor will ask the parents questions about the child's behavior. The second step is more thorough and may require doctors who have special knowledge. To diagnose older children, special education teachers at school may run tests. Then the child may be sent to a doctor.

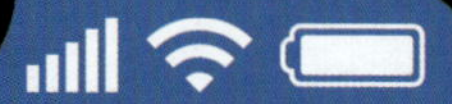

SYMPTOMS OF ASD

No two people with ASD have exactly the same symptoms. Symptoms of ASD are broken down into four categories: communication, social behavior, **stereotyped** behavior, and other behavior.

The following are just a few symptoms of ASD:

- Avoids or resists physical contact (social behavior)
- Talks in a flat, robot-like, or sing-song voice (communication)
- Flaps hands, rocks body, or spins self in circles (stereotyped behavior)
- Unusual reactions to the way things sound, smell, taste, look, or feel (other behavior)

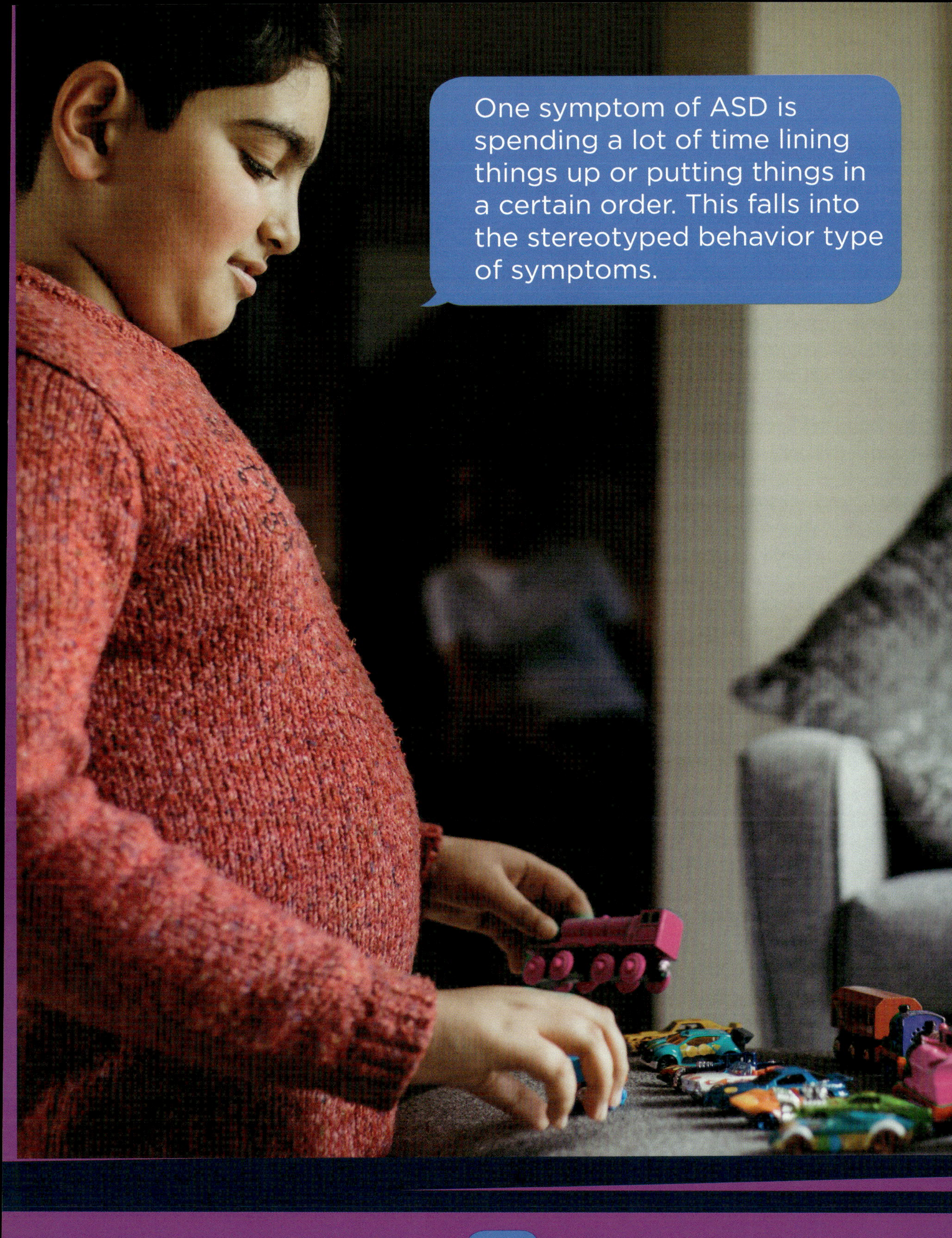

One symptom of ASD is spending a lot of time lining things up or putting things in a certain order. This falls into the stereotyped behavior type of symptoms.

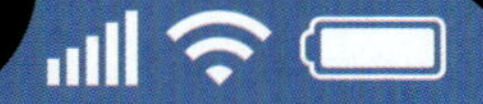

WHAT CAUSES ASD?

Scientists think a combination of a person's genes and **environmental** factors lead to someone developing ASD.

Genes are bits of **DNA** that control how a living thing looks and grows. Chromosomes are the parts of cells that contain the genes. If certain genes have a mutation, or a slight change, a person may develop ASD.

Stereotypes about people with ASD are often harmful. Many people with ASD lead successful lives.

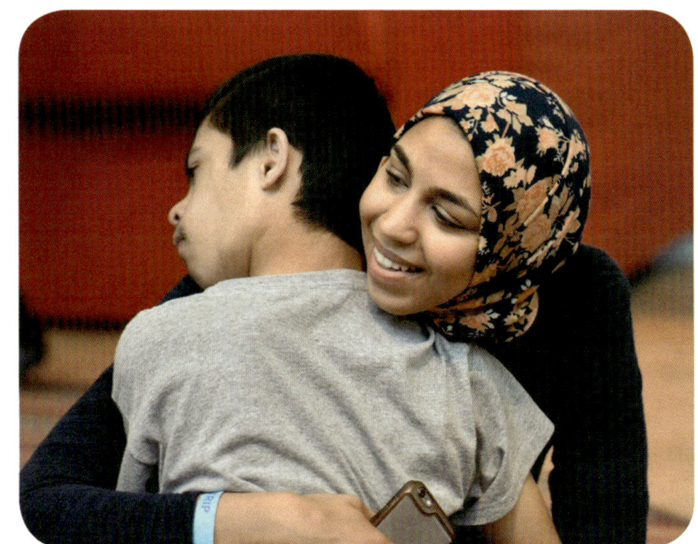

Environmental factors, such as infections, medications, air pollutants, or problems during pregnancy, may play a role in triggering ASD.

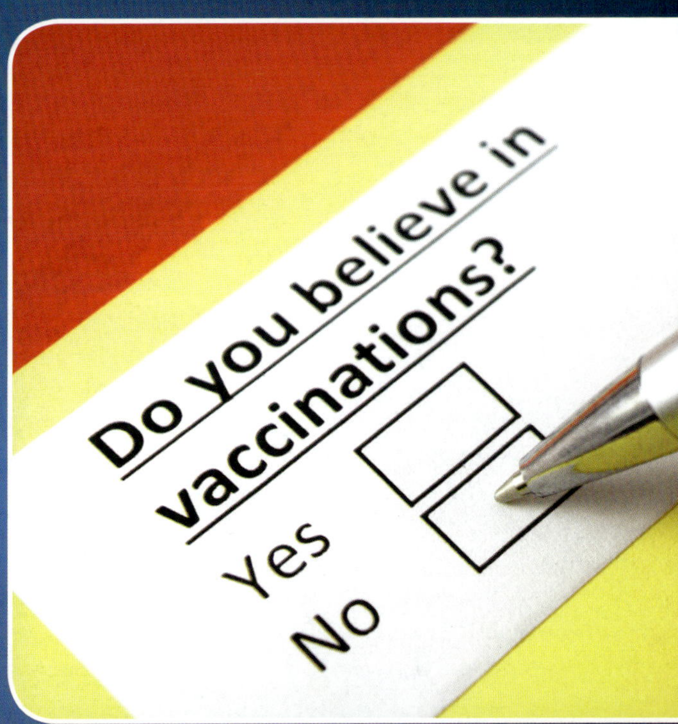

Fact!

In 1998 and 2002, Andrew Wakefield and other scientists published studies that said the measles, mumps, and rubella (MMR) **vaccine** causes ASD. As a result, many people choose not to have their children vaccinated. Wakefield's studies have since been **discredited**. Vaccines don't cause ASD.

ANTIVACCINE MOVEMENT

Wakefield's 1998 study linking ASD to the MMR vaccine started a dangerous movement of people who choose to not vaccinate their children. These people are called antivaxxers. Today, many people believe misinformation that antivaccine activists share on the internet. Children who aren't vaccinated can develop harmful diseases and can harm other unvaccinated children.

Chapter 2

Get the Facts Straight

My family and I live in Minnesota. Recently, a lot of people in Minnesota have gotten measles. For a long time, measles wasn't a problem in the United States. But a lot of people stopped vaccinating their kids. They were afraid their children would get ASD.

My sister Hillary has ASD. She's a wonderful person. But it hurts her feelings to hear that people choose to not vaccinate their kids because they think they'll get ASD. No one has ever died from ASD. But people die all the time from the measles.

Hillary wants people to get the facts straight. Recently, she talked to a group of parents at our school. She told them that not vaccinating their kids can harm them and other children too.

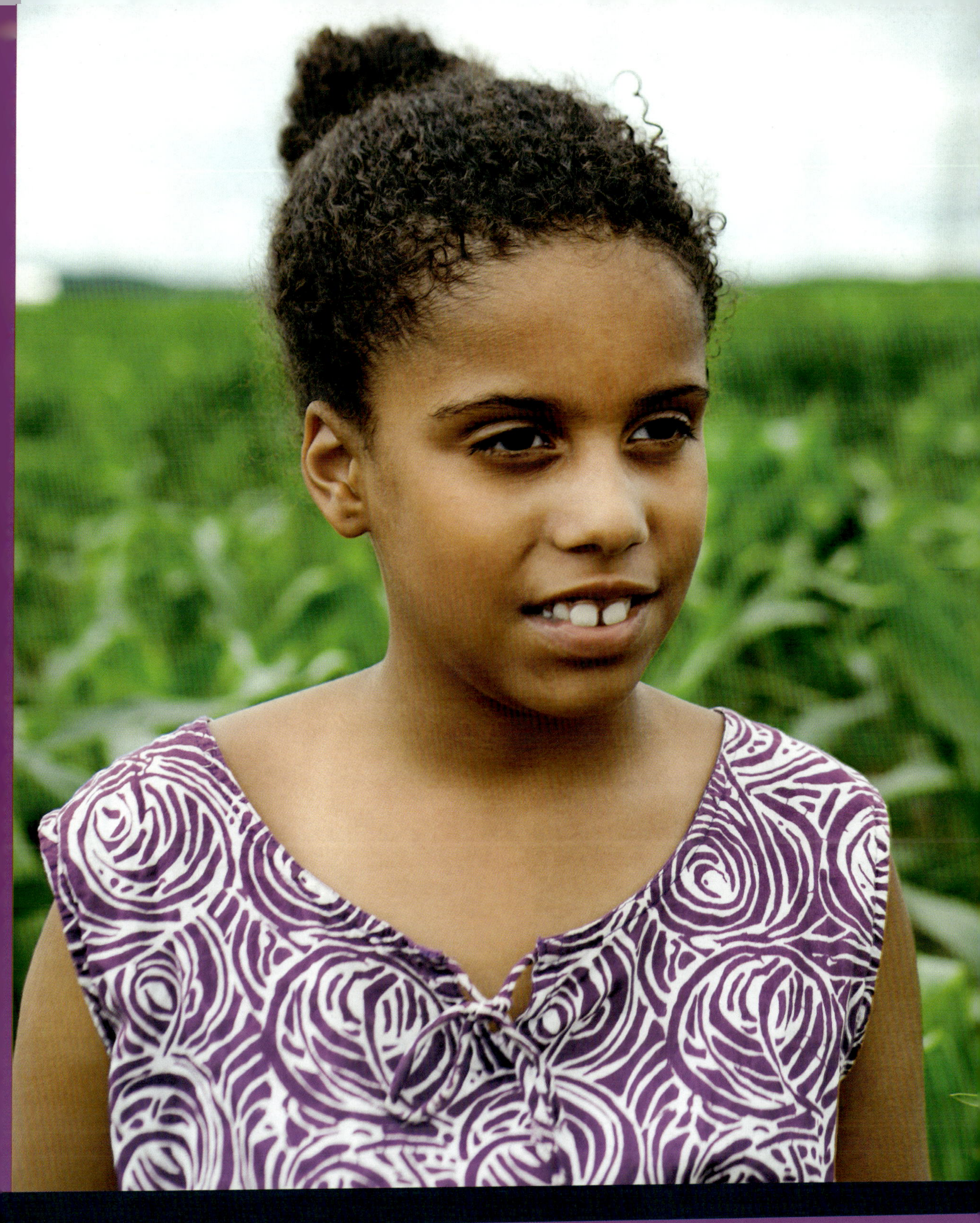

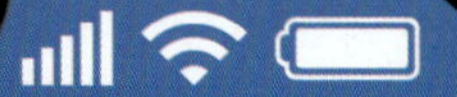

HOW IS ASD TREATED?

Because every person with ASD is different, this means their treatments are different too. The purpose of treating ASD isn't to cure the person. There isn't a cure for ASD. Treatments often make a person's ASD symptoms more manageable.

Some people with ASD have a hard time talking. A speech **therapist** helps people with ASD develop better verbal communication skills. They may help them communicate using hand motions or pictures.

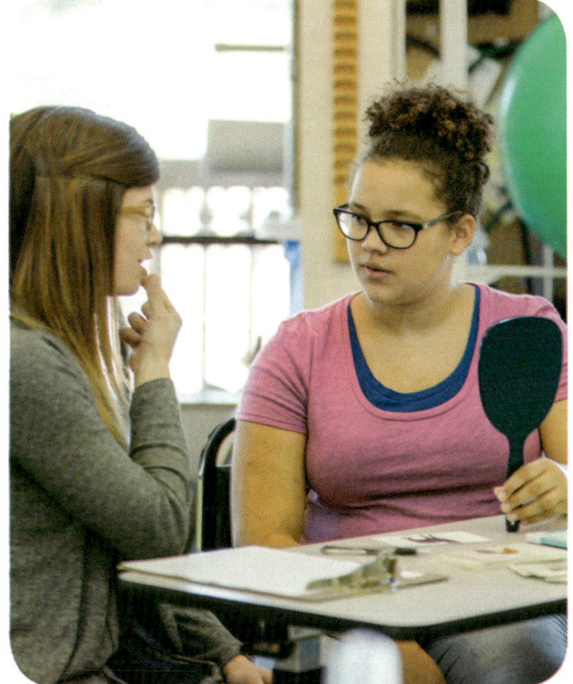

As soon as someone is diagnosed with ASD, they should begin treatment. The earlier someone's ASD symptoms are treated, the better their life will be. Doctors and other health care professionals will be able to find a treatment program that suits each person's needs.

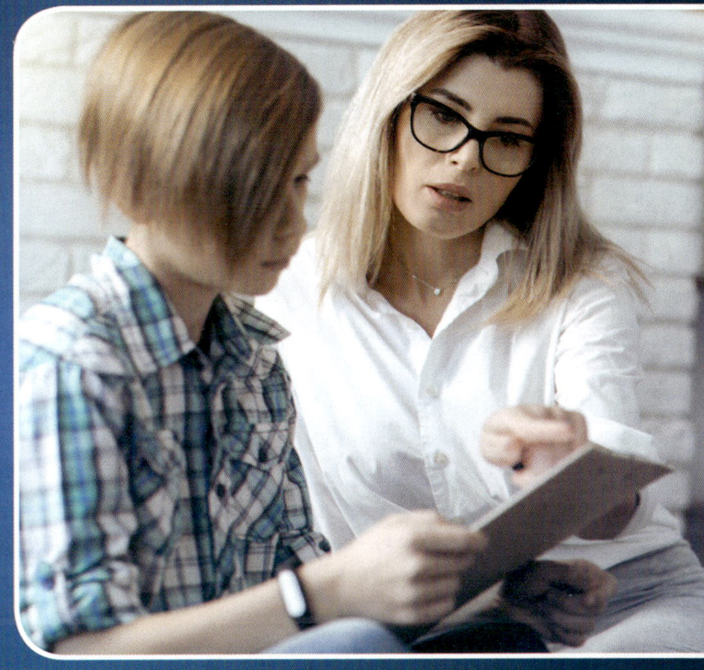

Fact!

It's important that people with ASD receive regular medical care. This includes routine checkups and dental exams. Sometimes it's hard to tell if someone with ASD is experiencing problems because of their ASD. It could be another health problem.

AT HOME AND AT SCHOOL

Many people with ASD receive treatments at home and at school. A therapist may come to their home to help them learn how to do things, such as eating and getting dressed, on their own. A therapist at school may help the person learn how to deal with sounds they don't like.

TREATING ASD WITH THERAPIES

A number of therapies can help treat ASD. Many of these therapies work to provide children with ASD with very routine care. They also get family members to take part in their care.

Some therapies help people with ASD get better at communicating, have better behavior, and have better social skills. Other therapies help family members learn how to help the person with ASD go about their daily lives and manage problem behaviors. People with ASD may also go to physical therapy to make their body stronger.

Fact!

Some people with ASD won't eat certain things. Other people believe certain foods make people with ASD's symptoms worse. However, science doesn't always support this. Before taking foods out of someone's diet, ask a doctor if that's the right thing to do.

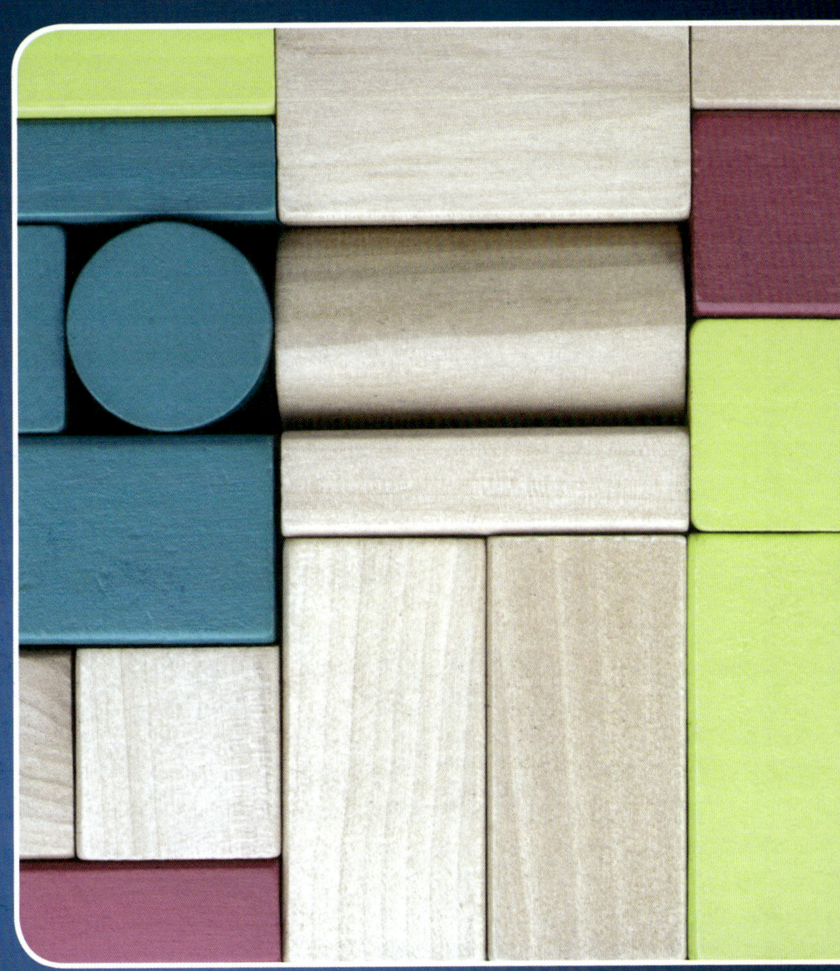

Different types of ABA help children with ASD work on different skills. One of these skills may be matching a pattern of colored squares.

APPLIED BEHAVIOR ANALYSIS

Applied behavior **analysis** (ABA) is used to help children with ASD learn new skills and put these skills to use in a number of areas of life. If they have good behavior, they are rewarded. They aren't rewarded for bad behavior. A therapist keeps track of the child's behavior to see if they're getting better.

TREATING ASD WITH MEDICINE

ASD's main symptoms can't be treated with medicine. Medicine treats symptoms of ASD, such as having attention problems, having too much energy, or having anxiety or depression. However, it's important to remember that medicine won't make someone's ASD go away.

Some people with ASD have other health problems. If someone has other health problems, they should speak to a doctor. Managing these problems can help people with ASD feel better. It can also make it easier for other ASD treatments to work.

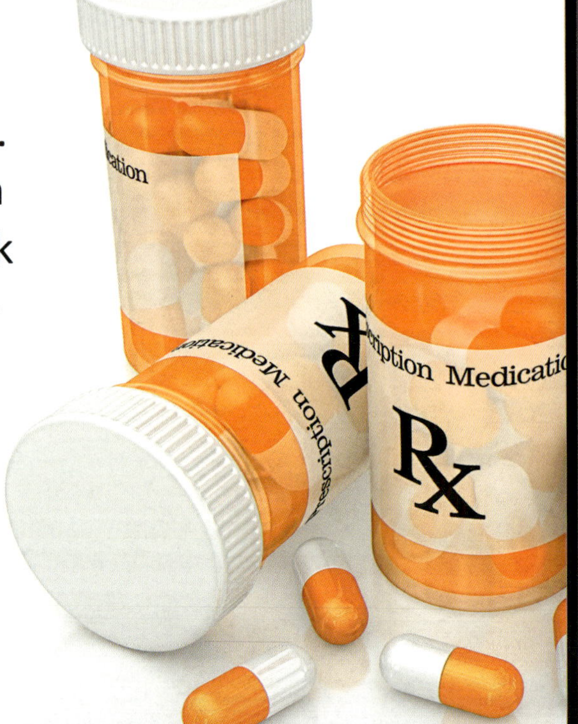

Medicines can help treat other health problems, such as **epilepsy**. If someone has ASD and epilepsy, treating the epilepsy with medicine can make the person's life better.

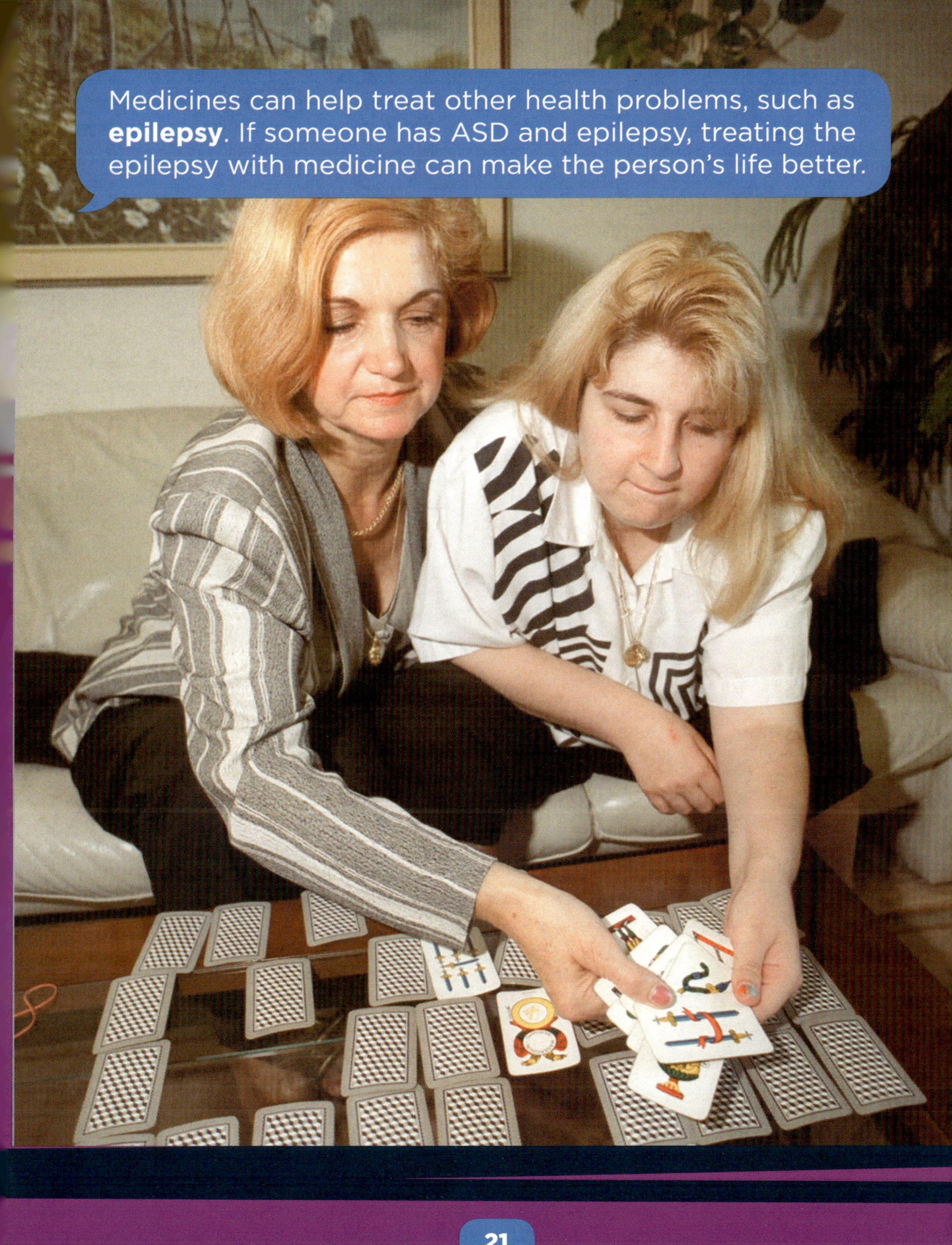

Chapter 3

Daniel Loves the Drums

Each week, I spend one of my free class periods helping out in the special education classroom. We do music therapy for the children who have ASD. Music therapy is supposed to help children with ASD work on their social and communication skills.

One of the kids in the special education room is named Daniel. Daniel doesn't talk. He also doesn't read or write. But he loves to play the drums. His face lights up when he plays and he smiles and laughs. On days when there is no music therapy, Daniel is less happy. Playing the drums is how Daniel communicates with me and his special education teachers. This year, Daniel has gotten much better at waiting for his turn.

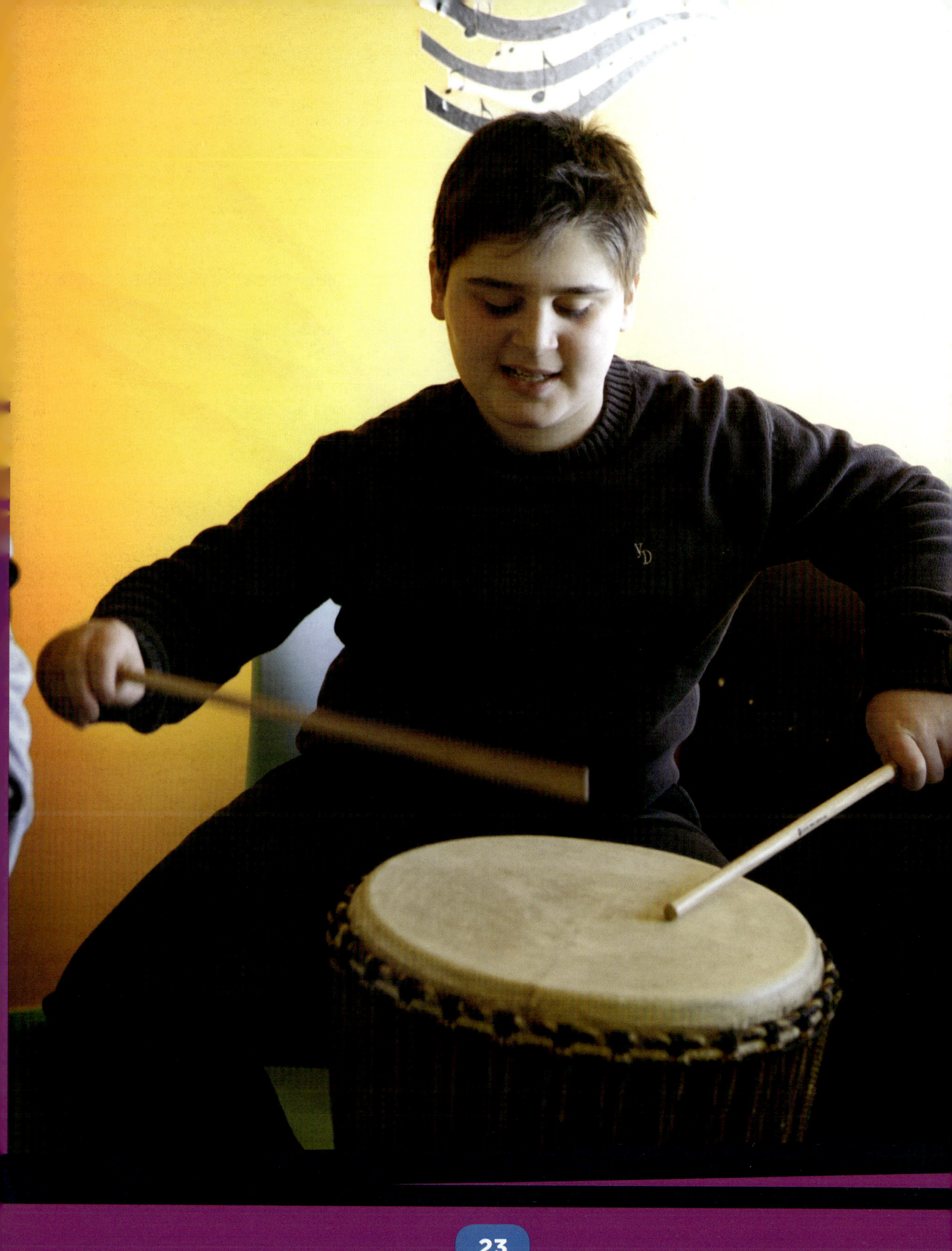

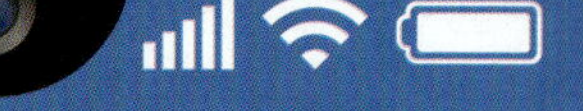

ASPERGER SYNDROME

Until 2013, Asperger syndrome was often used to diagnose people on the autism spectrum. Today, people aren't diagnosed with Asperger syndrome anymore. It's grouped into the diagnosis of ASD. However, many people still use this term.

The Netflix series *Atypical* is about an 18-year-old boy named Sam who has ASD. Sam's main goal is to find a girlfriend and become more independent.

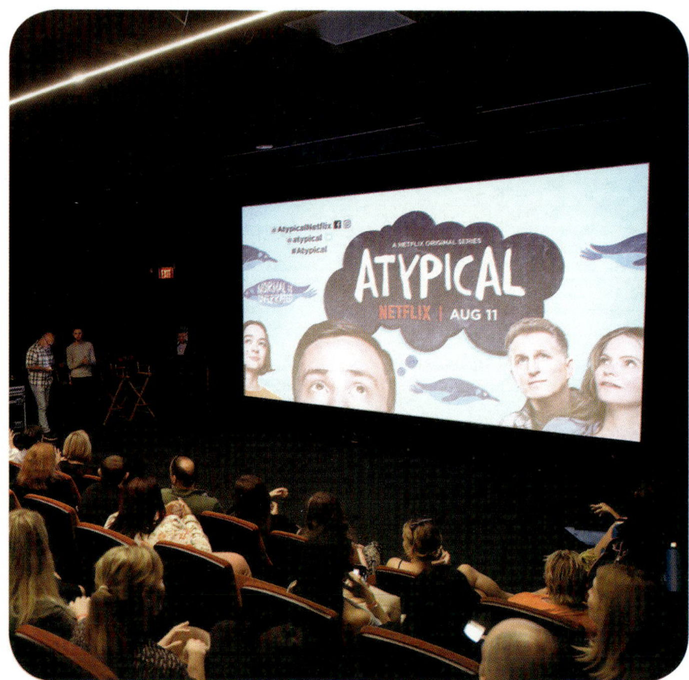

People with Asperger syndrome usually have better verbal, or spoken, language skills and intellectual, or mental, ability than others with ASD. They may become very interested in one topic and learn everything they can about it. People with this type of ASD may have trouble with things such as social skills and changes in routine.

Fact!

Asperger syndrome had a short history. In 1944, Hans Asperger, an Austrian pediatrician, first saw signs of the disorder in four young patients. It wasn't until 1994 that the diagnosis of Asperger syndrome made it into a book for doctors. It was added to the diagnosis of ASD in 2013.

VERBAL AND NONVERBAL SKILLS

Even though people with what was formerly called Asperger syndrome have good language skills, they may still have a hard time communicating. They may also have a hard time with nonverbal conversation skills, such as how loud they speak or how close they stand to others when they speak.

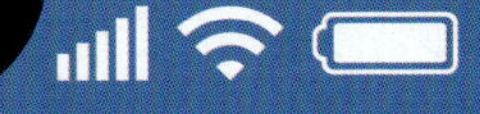

THE *DSM-5*

The *Diagnostic and Statistical Manual of Mental Disorders (DSM)* is the handbook health care professionals use to diagnose mental disorders. It tells them about different mental disorders and their symptoms. It has information to diagnose mental disorders. The original *DSM* has been updated four times, making the current handbook the *DSM-5.*

The American Psychiatric Association (APA) released the *DSM-5* in 2013. The *DSM-5* tells health care professionals what the signs and symptoms of ASD are. To diagnose someone with ASD, they have to have a number of the symptoms listed in the *DSM-5*.

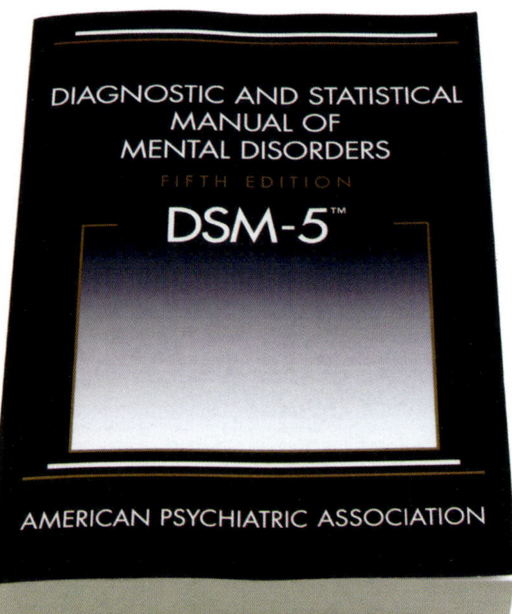

To be diagnosed with ASD, someone must show symptoms from early childhood. However, sometimes symptoms aren't reconized until later in life. The *DSM-5* makes it easier to diagnose people with ASD later in life.

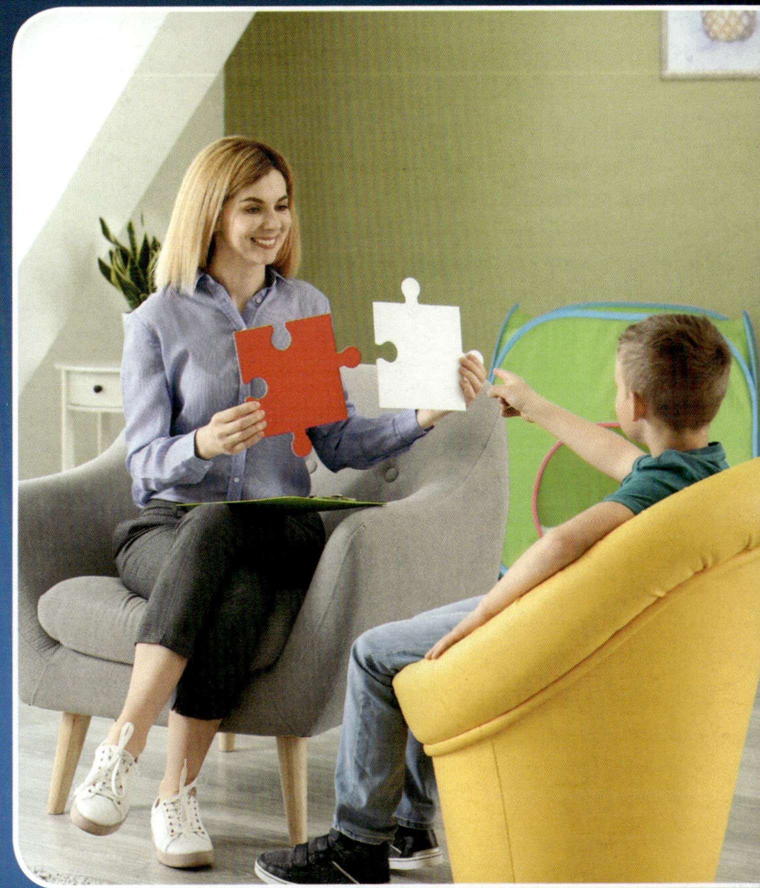

SOCIAL (PRAGMATIC) COMMUNICATION DISORDER

Social (pragmatic) communication disorder has similarities to ASD, according to the *DSM-5*. Someone with this disorder has a hard time with verbal and nonverbal communication. They may not take part in social situations. They may do poorly in school or have a hard time doing their job. A person can be diagnosed with this disorder if their symptoms don't fit with other disorders listed in the *DSM-5*.

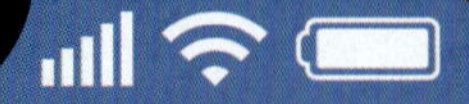

LEVEL 1 ASD

The *DSM-5* breaks ASD into three categories based on the level of severity. Each level of ASD requires a different amount of support. Support may be medical care, therapy, or help doing everyday things.

Someone with level 1 ASD would probably have been diagnosed with Asperger syndrome before the APA released the *DSM-5*. Without support, people with level 1 ASD have a hard time in social situations. They may also have a hard time making friends.

People with level 1 ASD don't need as much support as people with levels 2 and 3 ASD. They may receive behavioral therapy.

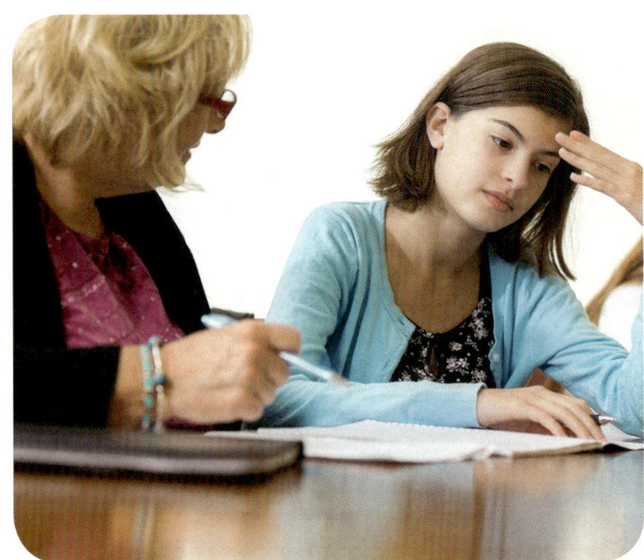

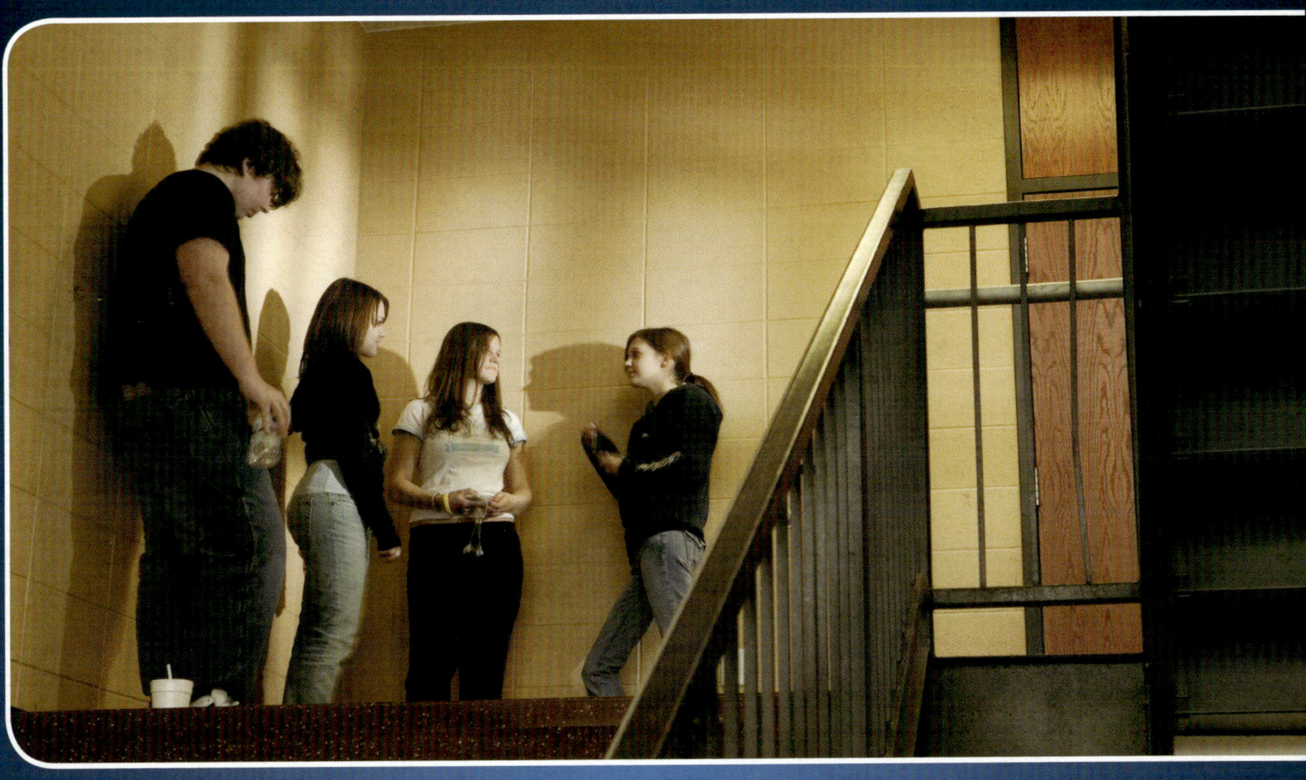

SYMPTOMS OF LEVEL 1 ASD

- Little to no interest in socializing with peers
- Hard time starting to talk to someone
- Hard time having conversations
- Hard time switching between activities
- Hard time planning and getting organized
- Hard time changing routines and behaviors

LEVEL 2 ASD

People with level 2 ASD require a lot of support. Support for people with level 2 ASD can be different types of therapies, such as sensory integration therapy. This can help the person deal with things they sense in their environment that bother them, such as flashing lights.

They have poor verbal or nonverbal communication skills. Without these skills, their daily lives are hard. Occupational therapy can help them develop skills that help them in their daily lives.

Sometimes, people with ASD have what's called a meltdown. This is when the person becomes overwhelmed by something. They lose behavioral control. The person may scream, cry, kick, or bite.

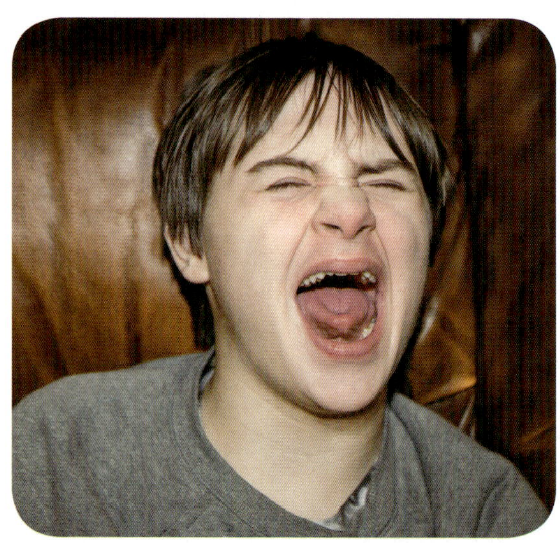

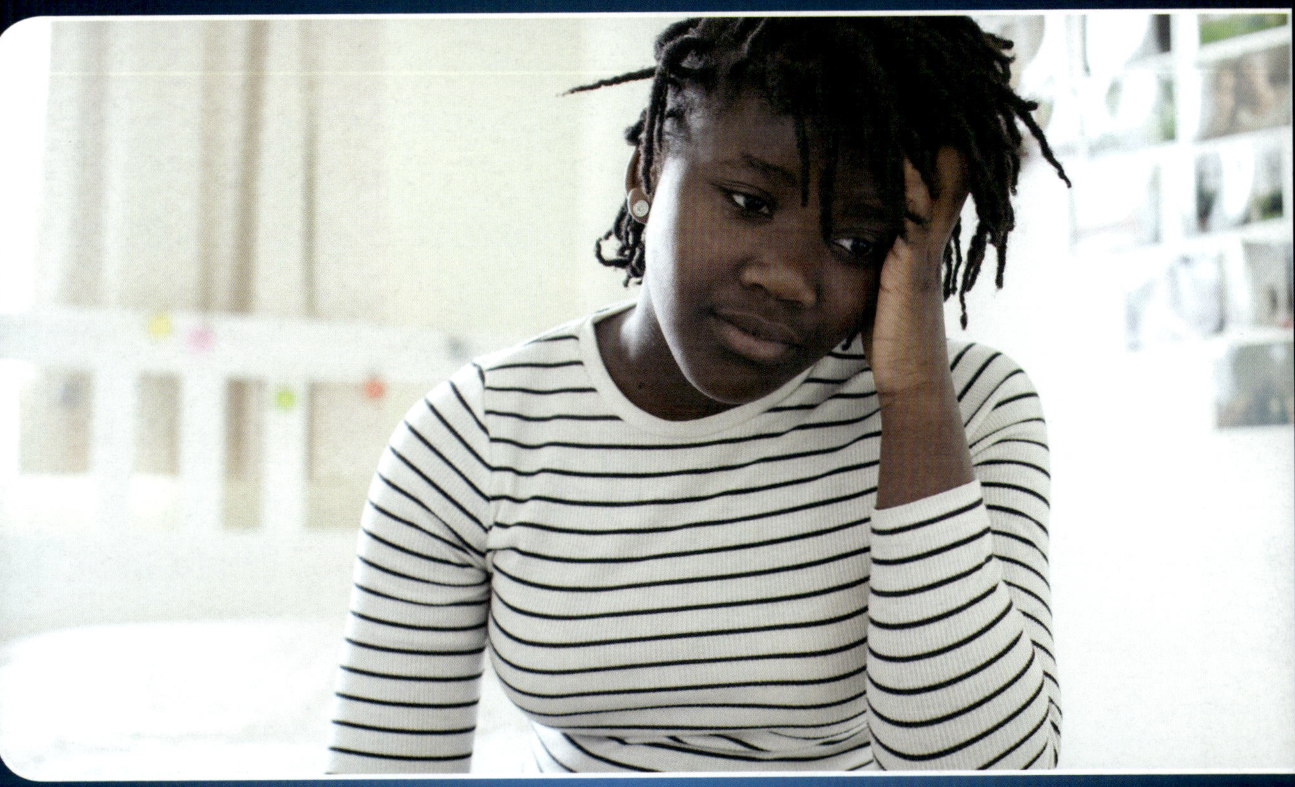

SYMPTOMS OF LEVEL 2 ASD

- Hard time dealing with changes in routine or environment
- Behavior problems or differences that strangers notice
- Few interests
- Trouble with verbal and nonverbal communication
- Simple means of communication
- Odd responses to social cues

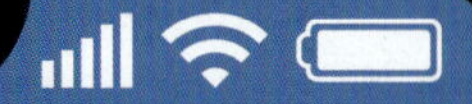

LEVEL 3 ASD

Level 3 ASD can be hard to deal with. People with level 3 ASD need even more support than those with level 2 ASD. They receive therapy more often to help them learn to communicate and do everyday things. Some people with level 3 ASD may need a caregiver with them at all times.

A person with level 3 ASD often has behaviors that keep them from doing everyday activities. They often do things over and over again, such as tapping on something or scratching themselves. This is called self-stimulatory behavior, or stimming.

Sometimes a person with ASD may feel far away from the people around them.

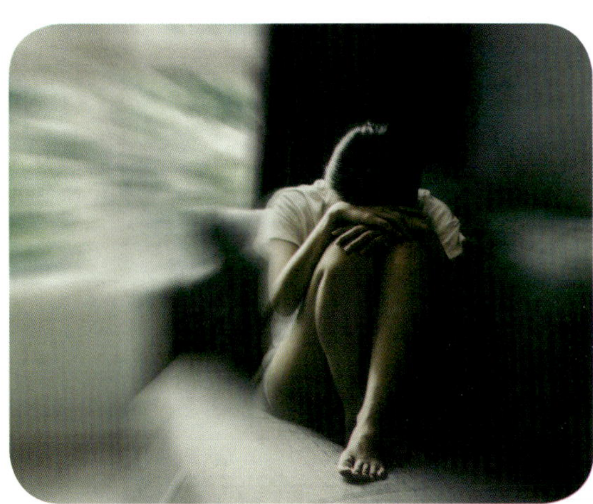

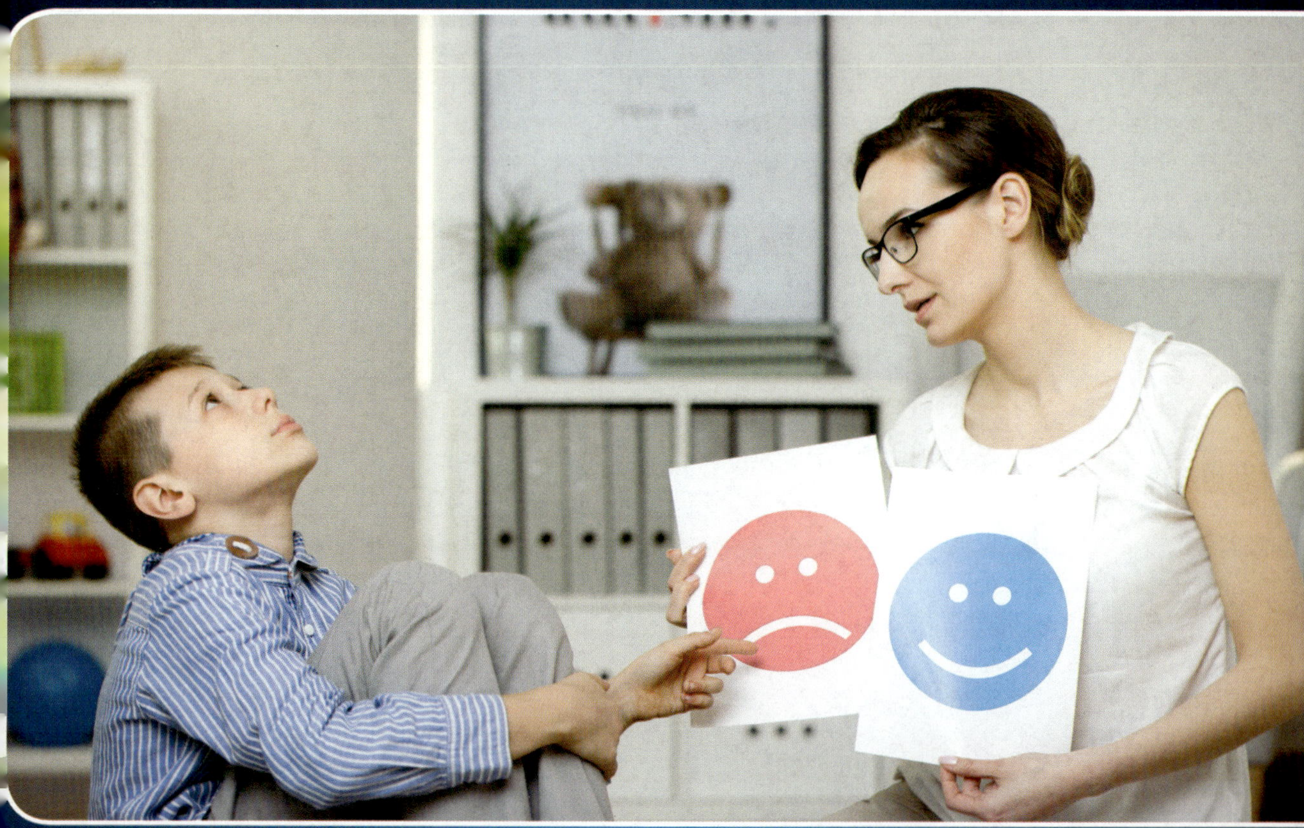

SYMPTOMS OF LEVEL 3 ASD

- A hard time changing behaviors
- A very hard time dealing with change
- Very low verbal and nonverbal communication skills
- Little response to social cues
- Getting upset at changes in activity or routine

Chapter 4

Walking for Jules

My cousin Jules has ASD. He's seven years old. He doesn't really know how to play. He loves to eat waffles. I wish more people understood ASD. Jules is nonverbal. This makes it hard for us to know what he's thinking and feeling. When he has meltdowns and stims, a lot of people stare at him and whoever's with him. They think he's weird.

Autism Speaks is a group that works to help people understand ASD. This year, we decided to raise money for Autism Speaks. We're going to do the Autism Speaks Walk in Austin, Texas, this spring. The money we raise will go toward funding **research** and supports and services for people with ASD. The goal of the walk is to improve the lives of people with ASD. That's why we walk for Jules.

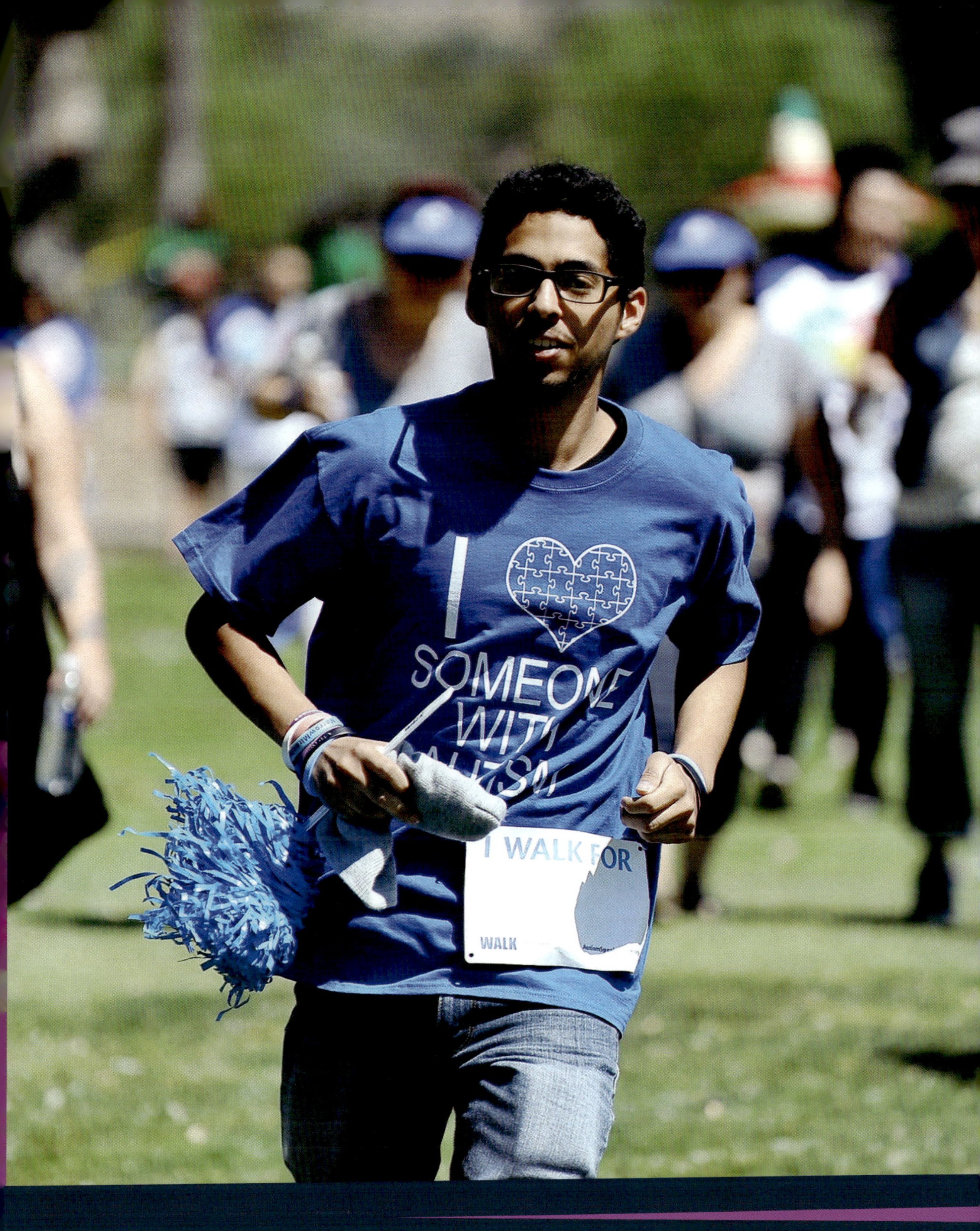
I
SOMEONE
I WALK FOR
WALK

ASD-RELATED CHARITIES

A charity is an organization that helps people in need. Different ASD-related charities put the money they receive toward different things. Some charities put their money toward finding a cure for ASD. Other charities may put their money toward helping people in a certain state or area.

Other charities put their money toward helping certain groups of people who have ASD, one type of therapy, or one type of research. Without charities, there may be fewer supports for people with ASD. There might not be as many research programs.

Resources

Autism Society of America
https://www.autism-society.org/
The Autism Society of America is a source of **advocacy**, education, information, support, and community for people with ASD and their families.

Autism Speaks
https://www.autismspeaks.org/
Autism Speaks is an organization that works to find solutions for people with ASD and their families. Money donated to Autism Speaks is put toward advocacy, support, and research.

The Organization for Autism Research (OAR)
https://researchautism.org/
OAR is an organization that uses research to answer the questions of people living with ASD. They spread new information to the autism community and aim to better the daily lives of people with ASD.

The Autism Speaks "Into the Blue" Gala on October 4, 2018, raised funds for autism research, programs, and resources.

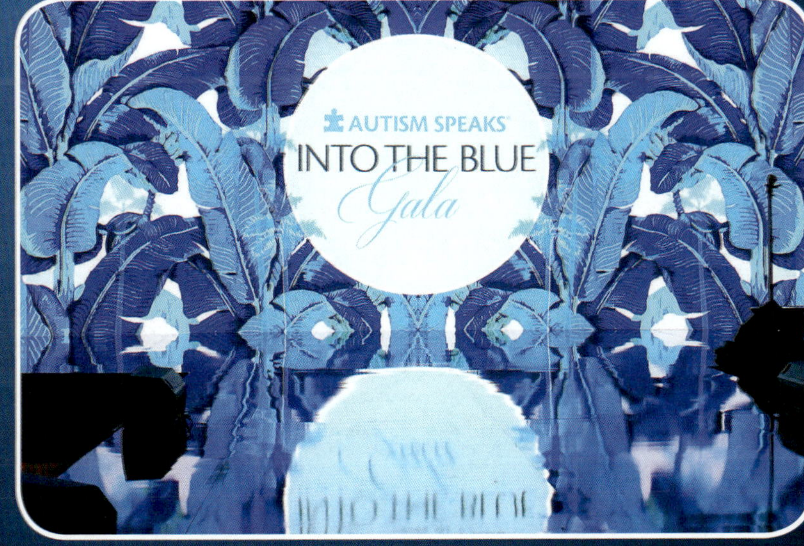

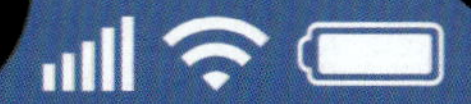

THE LATEST RESEARCH

ASD-related research is taking place all the time. In March 2020, researchers found that lowering levels of a **protein** called tau lessened autism-like behaviors in mice. Tau is a protein found in people who have Alzheimer's disease. However, lowering tau levels may help treat only some types of autism.

Another study has found that genes that help form a protective layer, called myelin, on tiny parts of the brain, called neurons, aren't normal in people with autism.

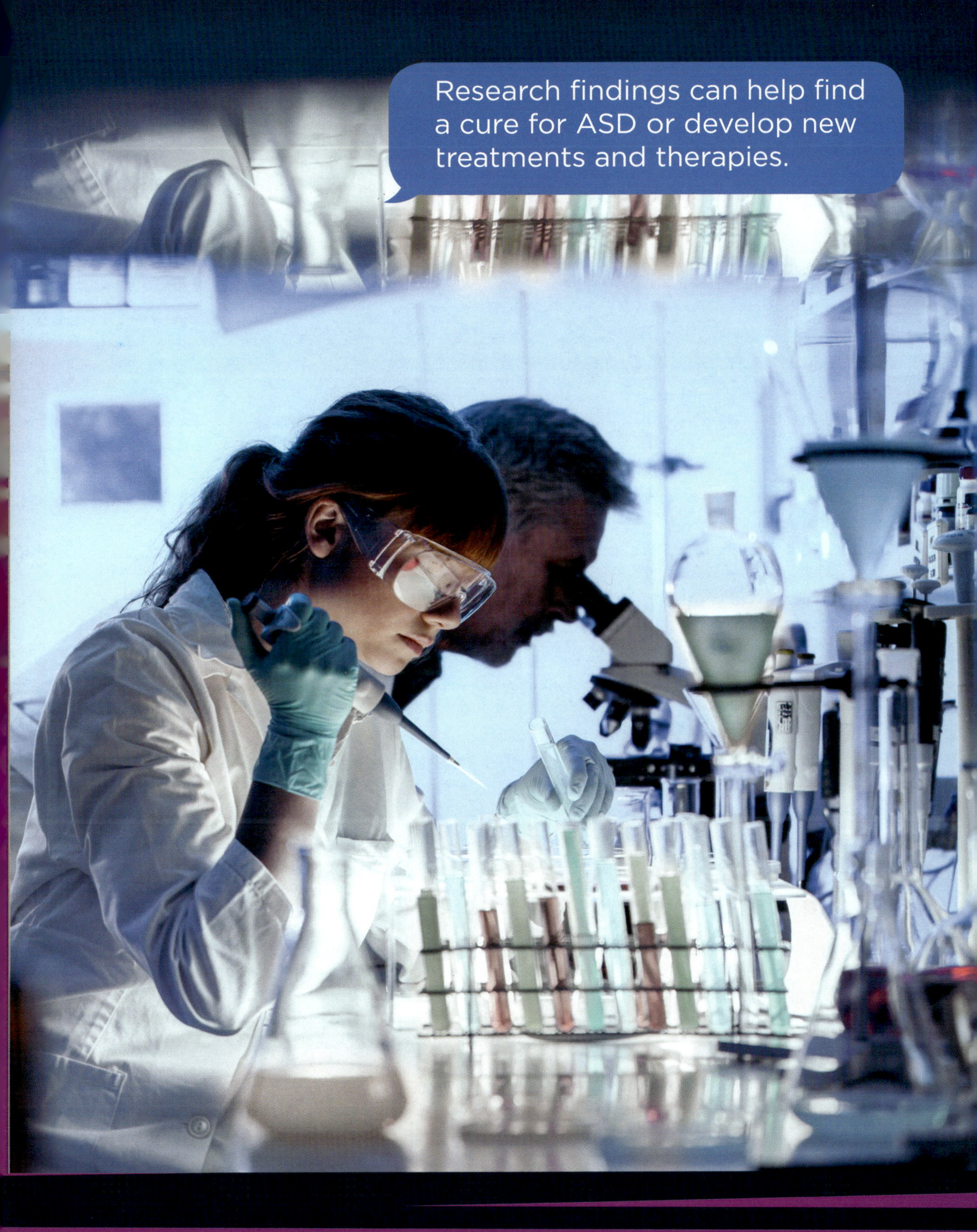

Research findings can help find a cure for ASD or develop new treatments and therapies.

LIVING WITH ASD

It's hard to know exactly what it's like to live with ASD. Everyone who has it is different. Normal activities can quickly become very **stressful** for people with ASD, though. Simply going to a café or playing on a playground can cause someone with ASD to experience sensory overload.

Some things people think of when they picture someone with ASD are being sensitive to lights, sounds, and touch. To cope with these sensitivities, people with ASD may shy away from being touched, rock back and forth, or flap their arms and hands.

Temple Grandin has shown that people on the autism spectrum can lead fulfilling lives. Having good support systems and ways to express themselves help.

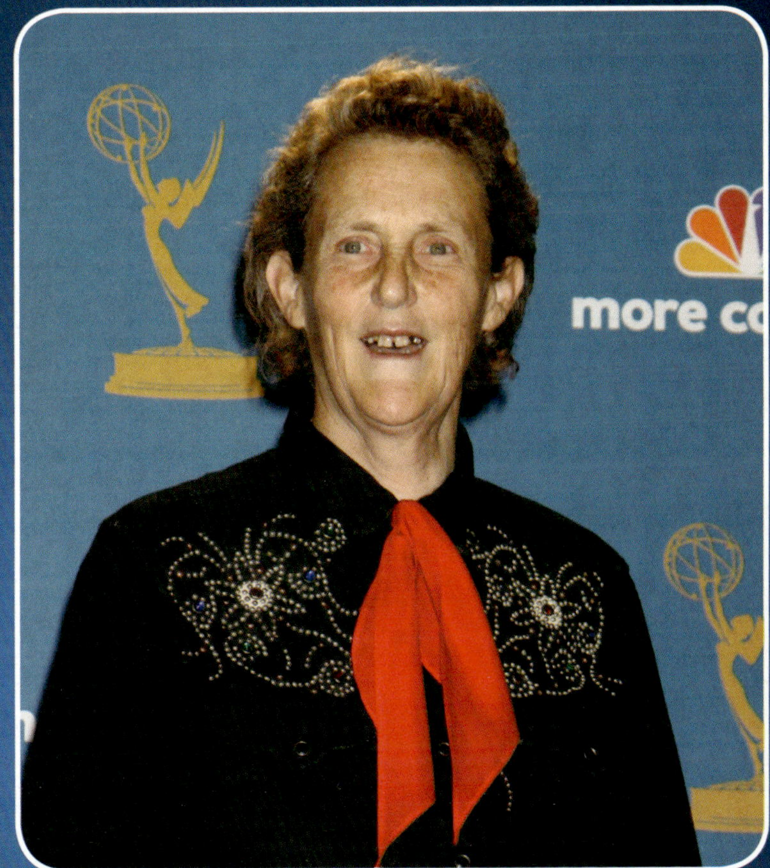

TEMPLE GRANDIN

Temple Grandin is a woman with ASD who has earned her PhD and works as a professor of animal science at Colorado State University. Her book *Emergence: Labeled Autistic* talks about what it's like to have autism. Grandin built a machine to squeeze her body to help calm her down when she was experiencing sensory overload. When she was very young, she screamed to communicate. Grandin understands things visually. This means she pictures them in her mind.

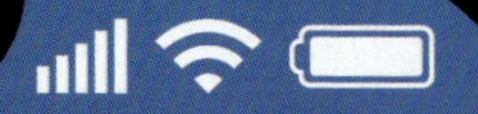

TRANSITIONING

It can be very hard for people with ASD to transition, or change, from one stage of life to the next. For example, transitioning from middle school to high school can be very scary. At some point, a person with ASD will need to leave school. At that point, they may need to search for a job or a place to live.

The Autism Society has resources for people with ASD who are transitioning out of school. These resources help people with ASD plan for life after school.

Fact!

It's hard for people with autism to find jobs. Even if they have college degrees, the application and interview processes are very stressful. About 85 percent of college graduates with ASD are unemployed. Integrate Autism Employment Advisors is a program that helps people with ASD get jobs.

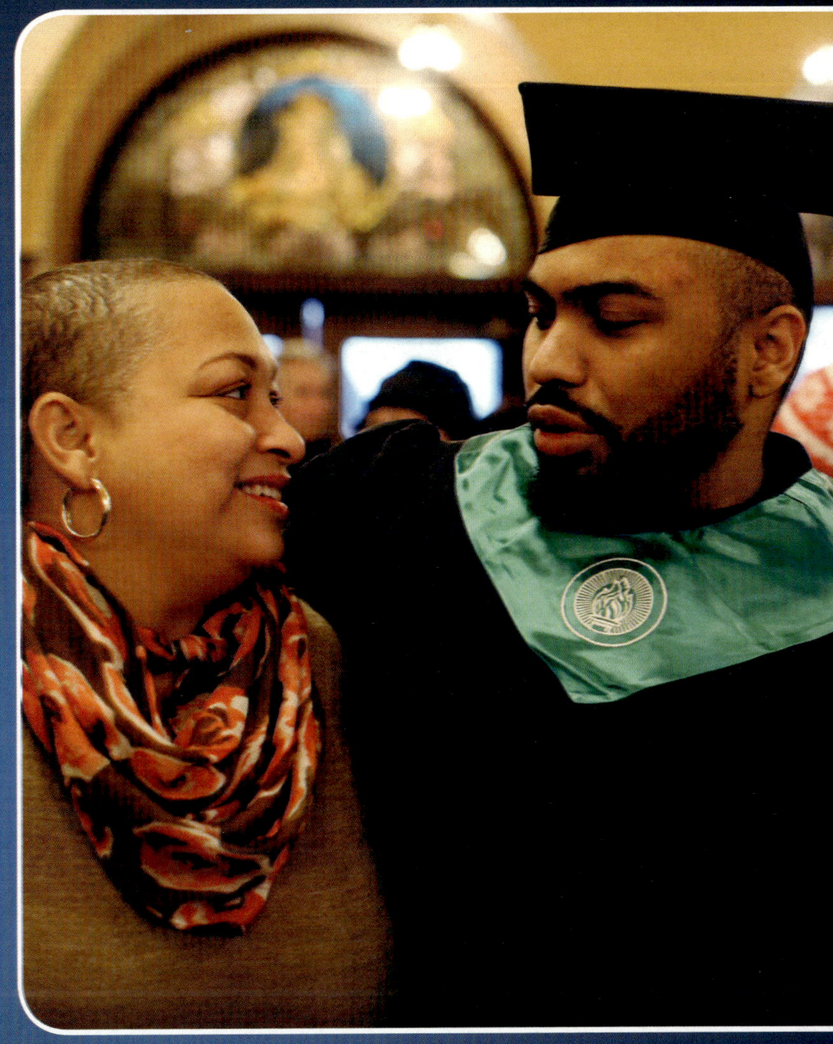

Having the right support is very important for people on the autism spectrum. With support, many people with ASD can graduate from college, get a job, and lead a fulfilling life.

OFF TO COLLEGE

Going away to college can be scary for people with ASD. Living with people they don't know, doing their own laundry, and waking up on their own are all unfamiliar things for many people with ASD. With the right support, people with ASD can transition to college life and learn to live independently.

Chapter 5

Helping Adam Prepare

My parents have been talking with Adam's guidance counselor a lot lately. Adam wants to go to the local community college next year. My parents aren't really sure what to think about that. They don't know if Adam will be able to handle it.

The guidance counselor told my parents that Adam can live at home while taking classes. He doesn't have to take a full class load either. He can go at his own pace. It's really nice to know that Adam has support.

I talked to Adam last night about what he wants. He said he wants to become a chef. I want him to follow his dreams. At the community college, he can take the classes he needs to get a job as a chef.

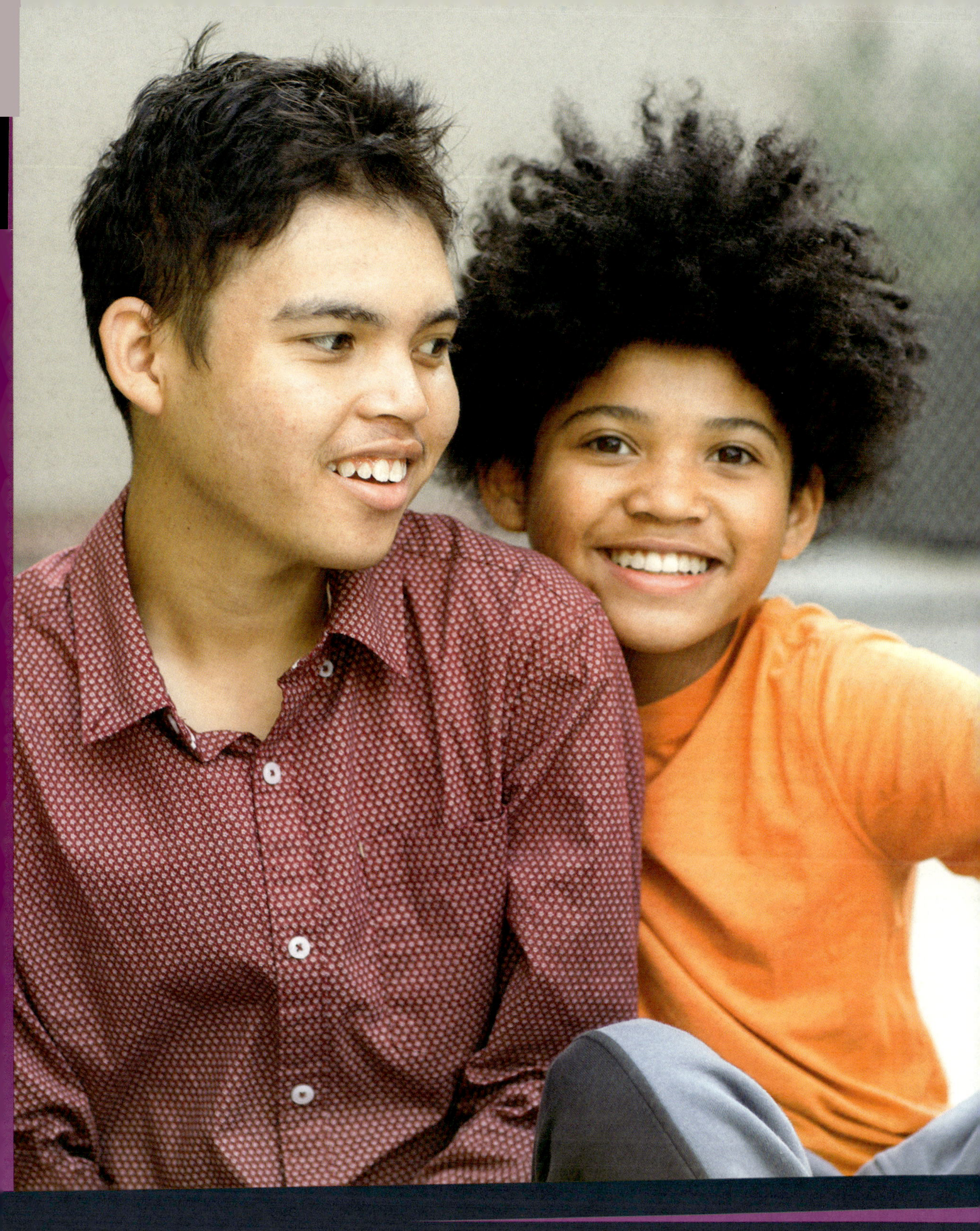

GLOSSARY

adapt: To change to suit conditions.

advocacy: Arguing for or supporting a cause or policy.

analysis: Close and careful study of something.

communication: The use of words, sounds, signs,or behaviors to convey ideas, thoughts, and feelings.

delayed: Moving or acting slowly.

developmental: Having to do with development, or the act of growing and changing.

diagnose: To identify a disease by its signs and symptoms.

discredit: To cause to seem dishonest or untrue.

disorder: A physical or mental condition.

DNA: A matter that carries genetic information in a plant or animal's cells.

environmental: Having to do with the natural world.

epilepsy: A disorder of the nervous system in which people have seizures.

fraternal twin: Either of a pair of twins that come from different eggs and may not have the same sex or appearance.

identical twin: Either of a pair of twins that come from the same egg and who look exactly alike.

protein: A substance found in foods, such as meat, milk, eggs, and beans, that is an important part of the human diet and is important for cells in the body to grow and do their jobs properly.

research: Careful study to find new knowledge.

routine: A regular way of doing things in a particular order.

stereotype: A commonly held idea about a group of people that isn't necessarily true.

stressful: Causing strong feelings of worry.

therapist: A person trained in methods of treating illnesses especially without the use of drugs or surgery.

vaccine: A substance that is usually injected into a person or animal to protect against a particular disease.

INDEX